POSTURE PAIN

Key Strategies to Stay Pain Free at Your Desk and in Life

Nicholas Gallo, PT, DPT

Disclaimer

The contents of this guide are based on my personal experiences as a licensed Physical Therapist and are for informational purposes only. This book does not constitute medical advice; the content of this book is not intended to be a substitute for professional medical advice, diagnosis, or treatment. Always seek the advice of a physician or other qualified health provider with any questions you may have regarding a medical condition. Never disregard professional medical advice or delay in seeking it because of something you have read on this website. Reliance on any information provided by this book is solely at your own risk.

Table of Contents

Introduction

I have written this in order to guide people with desk jobs who are struggling day in and day out with aches and pains. Most often, these small aches and pains are curable; however, the person who suffers from them will feel like they are not. I often hear things such as, "Oh I just have a bad neck," or "Eh, I'm just getting old." Having been a board-certified Doctor of Physical Therapy for some time now, I can tell you that these are poor reasons for a person's pain. Despite prior injuries and your age, you can always implement simple strategies to achieve a life of less discomfort – and in most cases, no discomfort at all.

One type of people that I commonly treat are those who "sit at a desk all day," or so they tell me. Believe it or not, in my experience, sitting for a prolonged period of time can put you in extreme discomfort and do more harm than other occupations. In most of the diagnoses I treat, there is often a culprit and a victim. What I mean is that I take into consideration the cause of a person's pain and the body part that is affected and starts to feel painful. In the case of desk jobs, I like to call sitting all day "the culprit" because it leads to a person's pain. Therefore, I like to refer to somebody's pain caused by sitting all day as "the victim" that is hurting due to the culprit.

In order for me to treat a person effectively, it is important that I treat the person as a whole. It is very simple to give a person stretch exercises and send them on their way; however, as a Physical Therapist I like to prevent these pains from coming back. As I commonly say, "Treat the culprit AND the victim." I want to teach people to sit in optimal postures and provide them with additional strategies that prevent discomfort. For the best results, I've treated the area that is hurting while providing people with strategies to keep them comfortable. Therefore, I would like to provide you with some tips and strategies that correct the daily routines causing these aches and pains. I hope that you will find this guide informative and easy to follow.

Before we begin, I would like to explain to you why bad posture at your desk can be detrimental to your well-being. When you engage in bad posture, you place your body in positions that it is not meant to be in. Doing this causes different areas of your body to hurt, and over time causes things to break down. I like to refer to a person's posture as the "foundation to the house." A house foundation is essential to how a house looks and how stable it is. If a house's foundation has issues, it compromises the structure of the house and becomes one hell of a problem (not to mention an expensive one). I want you to think of your body as the house and your posture as its foundation. Without optimal posture, you may be prone to detrimental injuries down the road. My goal is to prevent that with this guide.

I would like to share some research on this subject because that is a crucial starting point. In a study by Nejati et al., the subjects' working postures were compared to their forward-looking postures. The researchers concluded that the employees not only had defective postures but that improper posture was also more severe in employees that suffered from neck pain (1). I often use this study to show people the importance of posture correction because it can be applied to all office workers. I can also tell you that this is not the only study that shows the correlation between bad posture and pain. Therefore, I want to outline ways to improve your posture at work and during other activities, and give you key strategies to staying pain-free.

Finally, I would like to point out that I offer free educational videos showing exercises that improve posture on my YouTube channel Physical Therapy 101. This channel was started to provide free, to-the-point exercises to patients and practitioners. This channel is continuously being updated and provides a slew of information spanning several diagnoses, so please subscribe if you are interested. Supplemental information can be found on our website www.physicaltherapy101.net. Now, let's talk about posture!

1

Gravity Always Wins

Even though you have a desk job and it might feel like you need to sit at your desk all day, it is necessary to move around. I commonly tell people, "Gravity always wins." What I mean by this is that if you stay in one position for a long time, eventually gravity will pull you down towards the earth. Don't believe me? Hold your arm straight out in front of you. You should be able to do this without a problem. Now try to do this for the entire work day. I am willing to go as far as saying that nobody can hold that position for that long because eventually their shoulder will get tired. The same principle applies when you sit at a desk all day long.

As a person sits at a desk for a prolonged period of time, several things will occur. In no particular order, their shoulders become rounded and their head starts to fall forwards as well. Over time, this leads to increased tightness in the neck and chest musculature as they compensate to try and keep the head elevated, which results in pain. This also leads to weakness in the upper back musculature. When I see a person for this condition, their forward head and rounded shoulder posture is so bad that it is very obvious. Continuing down the body, a person may start to have wrist pain from a prolonged typing position. Our muscles can only support certain positions for so long before they start to get tired and cause pain.

Sitting for a long time also affects our lower body. Prolonged sitting causes a person's lower back to become rounded. Just like in the upper body, muscles try to compensate for this rounding of the lower back. Rounded back postures put extreme stress on a person's spine, especially their intervertebral discs. In fact, flexion-based postures are most commonly associated with disc herniations. Now, I'm not saying that sitting for a long time will result in a disc herniation. What I am saying, however, is that due to these bad postures muscles will compensate and eventually cause pain. Moreover, like in the upper body, muscles will fatigue and become tight, which also results in pain.

2

Set an Alarm Every 50 Minutes

So what can you do when you have a desk job and shouldn't sit all day? Do you just stand up? Yes, standing up is a great first step. I typically tell patients to stand up every 50 minutes; however, they often get engrossed with their work and forget. In my experience, after approximately the 50-minute mark, gravity begins to win and put people in a suboptimal posture. That is why I always suggest for a person to set an alarm so that they remember to change their position. Standing up combined with stretching your arms to the ceiling is a quick way to help fix some postural defects because it puts your body back in alignment. One thing I tell people to do in addition to standing up is to try and go for a walk. Not only does this help get you out of that bad posture, but it will also get blood flowing to your extremities. If there is one thing you take away from this guide, it should be this. Standing up and going for a brief walk is essential to preventing pain due to bad posture.

I also like to encourage people to buy certain things in order to increase their time standing. For instance, one product I own myself and really believe in is the standing desk. A standing desk is essentially a desk that allows you to stand while you do your work. There are many types of standing desks; however, they all serve the same general purpose. I cannot begin to tell you how many of my patients have got a standing desk and are very satisfied with their new piece of equipment. If I think a person can benefit from a standing desk, I usually ask them, "Will your employer pay for it?" Certain pieces of ergonomic equipment can be pricey, but employers may foot the bill in order to keep their workers injury-free. If this is not the case or you want to try something simulating a standing desk to see if it's for you, then you still have options. You can stack your computer monitor/laptop on boxes or books to the adequate height so that you can work while standing. (I will go over proper heights and distances for things like computer monitors and keyboards shortly.)

3

Treat the Culprit

First off, let's try to treat the culprit or the reason why people are so uncomfortable at their desk. After you've stood up for a while and gone for a walk, you sit back down at your desk. Take note of your posture. Did you just go back to those suboptimal postures I have been discussing? If you did, try to sit up and keep your ears in line with your shoulders. You should feel instantly that your neck muscles do not have to work nearly as hard to maintain this posture. The best way to visualize correct posture is imagining you have a line going from the top of your head through your body. In fact, that is how we learned about posture in graduate school. This technique is known as a "Plumb Line." We did this by literally attaching a string to the ceiling and standing or sitting next to it. We looked at each other from the side and were thus able to evaluate posture. This old-school but effective treatment is still used in a number of clinics to this day.

I've already told you the first step to correct posture and that is making sure your ears are in line with your shoulders by keeping your head back. This puts your head right on top of your spine and does not put additional stress on your body. Believe it or not, our head is actually pretty heavy. I like to ask patients to imagine their head is a bowling ball (they weigh approximately the same). Think of when you go bowling. When you select a bowling ball to use at the alley, you carry it to your lane as close to your body as possible because that requires the least work from your muscles. Now, if you carried the bowling ball further away from your body, it would be EXTREMELY difficult. The same principle applies to your head. The further out in front it is, the harder your body has to work in order to maintain that position.

Moving further down the body, the next thing to pay attention to is where your shoulders are located. Are they rounded forward? Are you shrugging your shoulders up to your ears? Most often, I find that people do a combination of both. Therefore, it's important, when you sit down, to keep your shoulders relaxed and down. Keeping the shoulders up and shrugged engages your upper trapezius muscles excessively and will lead to neck pains. In some cases, it can start to cause something known as a "tension headache." I usually give a cue to "Act like you're trying to put your shoulder blades into your back pockets." Additionally, if you notice rounded shoulder posture, I typically give people a cue to "Pinch your shoulder blades together as if you are trying to hold a pencil between them."

Now we get to the lower back. As I mentioned above, the lower back will start to round into that flexion-based posture when we sit for a long time. Sometimes this is just a natural process. When you feel it happen, it is time to stand up and go for a walk. However, there are times when this lower back flexion is extreme due to several different factors. First and foremost, it is of the utmost important that a person's chair is the correct height for them. A simple way to check this is to see if your knees are approximately 90 degrees with your feet sitting flat on the floor. In addition to the knees at 90 degrees, you want the angle of your hips to be 90 degrees as well. If the chair is too low, it results in the angle at the knee and hips to be less than 90 degrees. This will result in increased flexion at the spine. If the chair is too high and feet are not flat on the floor, the angles at the knees and hips are unable to attain 90 degrees as well. Therefore, in order to avoid the sensation of slipping out of the chair, a person will constantly engage their muscles to compensate. Why is this significant? As these muscles constantly work overtime, they begin to cause pain and discomfort. One good addition to your desk chair in order to prevent extreme spinal flexion is a pillow behind the lower back. This helps the lower back maintain the natural curvature of your spine and decreases the chances of it going into abnormal flexion.

Fortunately, in today's world most desk chairs are adjustable. Even if they are not, there are some strategies to still improve posture. If the chair is too high, you can simply place a book or box under your feet to raise the floor surface. If the chair is too low, you can raise the chair seat by sitting on an elevated cushion. Once you have set up your chair height correctly, I tell people to act like there is a string attached to the ceiling that is pulling them upwards. This tends to put them in a correct posture instantly.

4

Optimal Computer Station Setup

Now that I've briefly discussed chair height and how you should have your knees and hips at a 90-degree angle, it's time for the next step. Another huge component of proper posture at your desk is the computer station setup. The computer monitor, keyboard, and mouse positions are extremely important and should not be overlooked. Then there are also the other accessories that are used in the office, such as a telephone. I will go over some strategies of dealing with those as well.

Starting with the computer monitor, I always make sure the person's computer monitor is right in front of them. People in offices often put their computer monitors off to an angle, which should be avoided. This places a static rotational force on the neck and will lead to muscle imbalances and pain over time. If this is you, try your best to place the monitor directly in front of you. Once the monitor is directly in front of you, make sure the top half of the monitor is at eye level. This, coupled with the cue of imagining a string attached to the ceiling pulling you upwards, helps people maintain a good upright posture. If you do not have access to an adjustable computer monitor, you can implement some of the strategies I gave above to help adjust the chair height. If the computer monitor is too low, I suggest placing a book or box under the monitor to raise it to the ideal height. If it is too high, try the raised cushion method above, but make sure you keep your feet flat on the floor. One thing I do not really put much emphasis on is the distance a person's computer monitor is from their eyes. We were taught that approximately 2-2.5 feet is ideal, but as people have varying eyesight levels, I can only suggest that you play around with the distance so that you can both work pain-free and see well.

Moving down to the keyboard, it is ideal to have the elbows at 90 degrees with the keyboard at elbow level. Without me explaining why this is important, let's do an experiment really quickly. I want you to put your keyboard at a height that is too high for you. What do you notice? Usually, the wrists will compensate by going into additional flexion. Now try to type with the keyboard too low. In order to type in this position, your wrist goes into additional extension to compensate. Over time, either of these become extremely uncomfortable and will lead to wrist pain. If you do either one long enough, you might even notice numbness and tingling sensations because this position will begin to cause what is known as carpal tunnel syndrome. The name of this condition is based on the name of the wrist area that is being compressed, the carpal tunnel. You are compressing the nerve that passes through. In order to reduce compression in this area and allow the nerve to glide freely, it is important to have the elbows at

90 degrees and the keyboard at elbow height. This position allows the wrists to remain neutral and reduces the risk of wrist pain and/or carpal tunnel syndrome.

Now, let's head over to the computer mouse. To keep it simple, the mouse basically follows the same rules as the keyboard. You ideally want your elbows at 90 degrees and the mouse at elbow level. You can try the same experiment we did with the keyboard to feel why a mouse that is too high or too low would cause pain in the wrist over time. The mouse ideally should be right next to the keyboard. It should not extend past the keyboard or come closer than the keyboard. I like to use the visual cue of the computer keyboard width for a nice approximation of where the mouse should stay. Without sounding too corny, I like to call this area, "the mouse trap" because that is where you want the mouse to stay.

The desk phone is a very interesting piece of equipment that we also need to talk about. I find the desk phone interesting because there are so many variations to its placement. First off, if the phone is something you use regularly at your desk, it is smart to place it within reach. This might sound obvious, but I have noticed that some desks have things scattered all over the place. You want the phone within arm's reach if use it regularly to avoid having to bend and reach when you answer it. When treating someone who works at the front desk of a business for instance, I typically suggest that they use a wireless headset. These people are on the phone for the majority of the day and the wireless headset makes their life a whole lot easier.

If you only have access to a classic phone, be sure you use it in the best way possible. First off, I tell people to make sure they keep their elbow down when speaking on the phone. I tell people this because the more you raise your elbow out to the side while holding a phone to your ear, the more you are impinging your shoulder. Try this position for a second, put your hand to your ear like you are talking on the phone and now raise your elbow out to the side. You'll notice that the higher you go, the more difficult it is to hold it to your ear. Some people may actually start to feel shoulder pain. Additionally, its best to keep holding the phone to your ear with your hand and NEVER pinch it between your ear and your shoulder. I know that we are very busy and people like to multitask, but you may be on a call for a long time. The longer you are in that bad posture, the more of a toll it will take on your neck. For people who are on long calls and have to multitask, I usually suggest that they put the call on speakerphone if it's appropriate.

5

Ditch the Laptop and, If You Can't, Modify It

Laptops seem convenient because they can be taken nearly anywhere and make our work portable. However, they are responsible for extremely bad postures. Depending on its size, a laptop can cause a person to shift their entire posture just so that they can get a good view of the computer screen. The laptop is causing this because the monitor height and keyboard cannot be adjusted (unless there is a product out there that I am not familiar with). Fortunately, technology has come a long way, and now wireless keyboards and wireless mice have been invented. I tell my patients who work on laptops all day that I am a big proponent for getting these two items. Not only are they fairly inexpensive, but your body will thank you. You can purchase these two things and set them up just like I mentioned above. You do not necessarily need to spring for a brand new computer monitor because you can just place your laptop on a raised surface until it is at the ideal height.

I never noticed how bad laptops were for posture until I went to grad school. In grad school every person in our program got a laptop to help with classwork and assignments, and we were on them constantly. It was ironic because we were in Physical Therapy school and learning about bad postures and injuries from them, but when I looked around the room one day I noticed that nearly all of us had fallen victim to this! Fortunately, most of us were fine, but I could not imagine doing that at a job until retirement age. That is why it is imperative to make modifications to your laptop if you need one for work.

6

Mobile Devices

If I am going to give laptops a hard time, I absolutely need to include mobile devices too. There is a study by Jung et al. that looked at whether or not smartphone use affects posture and respiratory function. What they were able to conclude was that prolonged smartphone use can have a negative impact on a person's posture as well as their respiratory function due to this bad posture (2). I do not have much experience in dealing with a person's respiratory function, but this study supports my experiences when it comes to posture.

These days, almost everyone has a cell phone, and they can be horrible for your posture. They are also very commonly used at a person's desk in the workplace, so it is important for me to include them. Likewise, tablets are being used in a number of industries now and are owned by a large population of people. To share a real-life example, I was at an appointment the other day. While I was sitting in the waiting area, another person was also waiting on their appointment, and their posture was absolutely horrendous. If you look around a large group of people, you will most likely see what I saw. Hunched over, head forward, and shoulders extremely rounded to look at the screen. I know I'm also guilty of doing this, as most people are. However, because we use these devices so much, we really should try to use them in the most optimal posture possible. Mobile device use and bad posture has become so bad that I have treated a number of people for something I call "text neck." This is a slang term I use. Obviously, the act of texting is not always a person's pain; however, it is the position people fall into when gravity wins while they're on their cell phone or tablet.

The first step to stop having pain is something our parents have told us since we were young and that is, "Stop slouching." Sitting up straight when looking at your mobile device is nearly all you need to do in order to correct this, but a few other details should happen too. If you sit up straight and hold your cell phone too low, then you are creating a problem just like we had earlier with the computer monitor being too low. Therefore, I tell people to "Act like you are taking a picture." What do I mean by this? When we take a picture with our cell phone or tablet, we bring it up to eye level and have it right out in front. What people do not realize is that when you are doing this, you are putting the device in the ideal position for great posture! I'm realistic, I know you will not always do this when they're texting somebody or watching a show, but as long as you're conscious of it and make more of an effort to hold up your device, that is an immediate improvement. It's best to hold your device at that eye level I told you about for the computer monitor. If you use your phone or tablet a lot for work, try to treat them just like the laptop above. Purchase some wireless products you can adjust to a custom fit for better posture.

A lot of people also answer their phones in a suboptimal way . I want you to put your cell phone to your ear like you are answering a phone call really quick. Are you tilting your head to the side of your cell phone to bring your ear to the speaker? Is your elbow flared out to the side? Is your shoulder shrugged upwards? If you were to multitask, would you pinch it between your ear and shoulder? These are very common things I see and they should be avoided. While holding your cell phone to your ear, maintain the optimal neck posture I discussed earlier where the ears are in line with the shoulders. Try your best not to tilt to the side of the cell phone and keep your shoulders down instead of shrugging them upwards. I know that during busy days you will most likely need to multitask while on the phone, so I will provide the following strategies. First off, if it is appropriate, put the conversation on speakerphone for the brief time you need to multitask. This will free up the hand, head, and neck so you can remain in good posture. If you are uncomfortable doing this, you can purchase a headset or a hands-free addition. Finally, instead of flaring the elbow out, try to keep it tucked into your side like you are trying to touch your elbow to your ribs. You should feel that having your arm in this position is not only easier to hold up your cell phone, but it is also much more comfortable.

7

Treat the Victim

We have now successfully set up our workstation and treated the evil culprit. Once you have done this and have become more cautious about engaging in bad postures, you have already taken the first step towards recovery. Now I want to provide ways to treat the victim, which would be certain aches and pains people have due to being in bad postures over time. In my experience, the pain can be treated with some simple exercises and stretches. In order to make it easier on you, I would like to share ways to perform them at your desk. Does the research community support such programs in order to help with posture correction and musculoskeletal pain? You bet it does. In fact, a study by Kim et al. focused on this exact subject. They concluded that people with pain in their shoulders, middle back, and lower back had a SIGNIFICANT decrease in their pain levels when implementing such a program (3).

The issue that I often run into is that people do not know which exercises to do. Therefore, I will outline some key exercises and stretches that have worked for my patients in my clinical experience. One important thing I want to tell you before I begin is that it IS possible to overstretch a muscle. What I mean by this is that you can stretch muscles too hard and hurt yourself. Therefore, it is important that you perform the stretches through a pain-free range and that you don't stretch too strenuously.

Let's keep the same trend as before and start with the neck. I do not want to bore you and go too in depth with human anatomy, but in my experience, there are two key muscles that cause pain in the neck. One is known as the Upper Trapezius muscle, of which you have one on each side of the neck. You have used this muscle many times throughout your life but may not have known it. It has several functions, but when you shrug your shoulders, you are engaging both of them at the same time. Over time, this muscle becomes overworked and can cause neck pains. A great way to stretch this muscle is to start off by facing forward and keeping your head straight. Now hold on to the bottom of your chair with one hand and tilt your head the opposite way. For example, take your left hand and hold the bottom of your chair. Now tilt your head to the right, you should feel a big stretch in the left side of your neck, effectively stretching your left Upper Trapezius muscle. Now try it on the other side. You should feel a stretch on the other side of the neck. If you do not feel much of a stretch, you can use your other hand to pull your head into a more stretched position, but remember to NOT overstretch. For this stretch, I tell people to hold for 30 seconds and to perform it 3 to 4 times on each side.

Another important muscle in the neck that causes pain when it becomes tight is known as the Levator Scapulae. Like the Upper Trapezius, you have one on each side of the neck, so it's important to stretch them both. Like the previous stretch, start by facing forward and holding onto one side of your chair. Now, while facing forward, rotate your head slightly away from this arm and touch your chin to your chest. In order to stretch your left Levator Scapulae, hold on to the bottom side of your chair with your left hand and rotate your head slightly to the right. Now touch your chin to the right side of your chest. In order to stretch your right Levator Scapulae, perform the process on the other side. Remember to not overstretch. I also tell people to hold this stretch for 30 seconds and to perform the exercise 3 to 4 times for each side.

These muscles also play a role in rotating the neck, so I advise people to stretch them this way. Start by facing forward. To begin stretching the left side of the neck, begin by slowly turning your head to the right. If you already feel a stretch, you can hold your position for 30 seconds and perform it 3 to 4 times. If you'd like to provide some overpressure in this position, you could do that by using your right hand to push your left cheek to further take you into more rotation. Once you stretch the right, perform the stretches on the left side.

A great way to stretch several muscles in the back of the neck is as follows. While facing forward, let your chin fall to the center of your chest with your mouth closed. The mouth closed cue is important because I often see people misunderstand and try to open their mouth to reach their chest! You can provide some overpressure in this position by placing both hands on the back of your head and pulling the head down. You should feel a stretch on both sides of the back of your neck. Hold this stretch for 30 seconds and perform it 3 to 4 times.

Finally, we must stretch the muscles in the front of the neck. To do this, simply look up at the ceiling. With this position you should feel muscles stretching in the front of the neck. Here you are placing your neck into extension and I want to make it clear that it is NOT recommended to provide any overpressure here. Placing your neck into extreme extension can cause nerves to be pinched; therefore, I do not recommend that with this one. Like all prior stretches, try to hold this stretch for 30 seconds and perform it 3 to 4 times.

The next exercise I want to go over is called a chin tuck. We essentially performed this exercise earlier, when I told you to place your head in the center of your spine instead of forward, but I'd like to go into a little more detail. This exercise is important because it will start to strengthen and build endurance in the postural muscles. This exercise can be done anywhere and, once perfected, can be extremely beneficial. To start, just like before bring your head back to where it is directly over your spine and your ears are in line with your shoulders. Now from here, try to tuck your chin downwards. A cue I like to give people is to try and create a double chin. Everybody wants to prevent the double chin look, but in this case it is necessary! You will feel your muscles working in the neck to try and hold this position. Try to hold this position for 5 seconds and perform 30 repetitions. If you cannot perform this many repetitions right away, then that is completely fine. Try to build up to 30. If people are still struggling to maintain the correct position, I often suggest that they use a mirror so they can visualize themselves. If you don't have a mirror at your desk but have your cell phone, use the camera to visualize yourself.

Now I want to move further down the body and address the rounding shoulder posture. Usually, rounded shoulders are caused by weakness in the upper back muscles and tightness in the chest muscles. Therefore, I will begin by giving you a basic upper back exercise. The exercise I like to give people is known as the scapular squeeze. It is called that because you are simply squeezing your shoulder blades, anatomically known as your scapulas, together. The best way to perform this is to stick your chest out while squeezing those shoulder blades together. If it is tough to visualize, I tell people to "Imagine there is a pencil between your shoulder blades and you want to hold it between them by squeezing them together." It is important to try and hold this position for 5 seconds and progress up to 30 repetitions like the chin tuck exercise.

Let's talk about stretching the chest muscles. In my experience, the best way to stretch these is to use a doorframe. I like to discuss this stretch with people because I often see it done INCORRECTLY! First off, go to the doorframe and stand close in front of it. Now pretend like you are doing the "Y" in the song YMCA and put up both arms. Now walk into the doorframe with your arms touching the doorframe and lean in. As you are doing this, did your head just fall forward? That is the most common mistake I see. To get the maximum benefit of this stretch, it is best to keep your head in the good posture I have been discussing. Hold this stretch for 30 seconds and perform 3-4 repetitions. If you want to stretch your chest in different ways, try lowering your arms like you are mimicking a field goal post and repeat the same stretch. If you are able to, you can also lower your arms further to stretch different sections of the chest muscles.

The next stretch I particularly like because it is effective and can be done very easily at your desk. You might have even performed this stretch in the past and not even realized it. I hinted at this stretch earlier by telling you to do this when standing up, but it will accomplish the same goal when you're sitting down, so you can choose which option you prefer. Start by putting both arms above your head and putting your hands together. Now lace your fingers together and turn your palms upward. Now push your hands towards the ceiling. You may already begin to feel a stretch in this position. If you want to stretch the right side, tilt your body to the left and hold this position for 30 seconds. Try to perform this 3-4 times. Perform this stretch vice versa in order to stretch the left side.

As we move on to the spine, there are several different exercises we can perform to help posture. I went over the problems with staying in a flexed posture while sitting all day, so I'd like to begin with a great stretch to put your lower back into extension. The best way to do this is with the exercise known as a prone pushup. The first step is to lay prone on the ground, like you are about to do a pushup. When people first attempt this stretch, I tell them to first lie on their stomach with their hands under their forehead. The progression begins with placing your elbows under your shoulders and pressing up. You will press up, hold it there for 5 seconds and let your body back down onto the floor. Try to perform 10-15 repetitions. Now this stretch will become easier, and you will want to progress to a more difficult one. In order to do this, instead of having your elbows in contact with the ground, put your hands in contact with the ground. I tell people to push up until their elbows are bent and then go back to the floor. The toughest position for this stretch is when your arms are completely locked out and your lower body is resting on the floor. It is very important to not let your hips raise off the ground as you push upwards. Also, people tend to shrug their shoulders up as they are doing this stretch, which is a bad idea. It is important to keep your shoulders and hips down throughout the entire motion. If you are unable to lie down at work, I suggest performing this exercise standing up. The best way to do this is by placing both hands on your lower back and pushing them forward. Simultaneously, I tell people that they should be looking at the ceiling.

Commonly, tight hip musculature such as the Gluteals tends to result in the spine becoming flexed and, coincidentally, causes back pain. For those who do not know, your Gluteal muscles are most often referred to as your butt muscles because of their location. You can very easily do a great gluteal stretch while sitting in your chair. In order to stretch your left gluteal musculature, first cross your left leg over your right. You will know when you are doing this correctly when the outside of your left ankle is resting on your right thigh. If you notice that your left knee is high in the air while in this position, push it down with your left hand. You want to try and get your leg parallel to the ground while in this position. I have people hold on to their left ankle with their right hand in order to keep it in place. If you have not done this stretch before, you may already feel tightness. If you do, then hold it for 30 seconds and repeat for 3-4 repetitions. If this is not stretching you enough, sit up, keep your back straight, and begin to lean forward. You will not have to go very far before you start to feel a stretch in your gluteal muscles. When you have stretched your left side, repeat the above process on the right.

Another muscle that causes the lower back to round and will tighten after prolonged sitting is the Psoas muscle. The Psoas muscle has several functions; however, it is most commonly associated with being a hip flexor. This is an important muscle for lower back pain because it attaches from the front of the thigh to the lower spinal column. When I treat a person that comes to me with lower back pain, this muscle is more often than not the cause of it because it is often overlooked. The way this muscle is stretched is by getting down into a lunge position. I usually tell people to "Imagine you are going onto one knee to propose to somebody." While in this position, maintain a straight back and push your front knee forward. In order to stretch your left Psoas muscle, go onto one knee with your left knee touching the ground and your right foot making contact with the ground out in front. Maintaining contact with ground, push your right knee forward, making sure you keep your lower back straight. You should start to feel a stretch in the front of your left thigh. If you do not, try lunging out further and repeating the same steps. Like the other stretches it's important to try and hold it for 30 seconds and perform 3-4 repetitions.

Another great lower body stretch you can perform at your desk is the hamstring stretch. Your hamstring muscles are located in the back of both thighs and can be stretched in a number of ways. The easiest way is to maintain your leg as straight as possible and to place it on a raised surface in the seated position. You can vary the intensity of this stretch by changing the height of the surface that your leg rests on. As you place the leg on a higher surface, the stretch gets more intense and vice versa. Play around and see at which height you can maintain a straight leg with no bend in the knee. If you feel like this is not stretching you enough, lean your trunk forward maintaining a straight back. Try to hold for 30 seconds and perform 3-4 repetitions. As this stretch becomes easier, the best method is to just raise the surface your leg rests on until it is the same height as your chair. Once this becomes easy, this same stretch can be performed standing with the same progression. Begin with a low surface and then progress until your leg is resting parallel to the ground. A way I like to progress this stretch even further is by having a person lay on their back. Place a strap around your ankle (this can be a stretch strap or something such as a dog leash or a belt). Maintaining the leg straight, pull it up until you feel a good stretch in the back of your thigh. I also like to suggest the person bends the other leg and places the foot flat on the floor to help protect the lower back and prevent pain.

Finally, let's move on to the ankles. Your ankles and/or feet may begin to hurt throughout the day, so I want to include some stretches here for that. A good way to get your ankles moving while sitting is actually fairly easy. To start with the left leg, begin by straightening your left leg out in front of you. Now point your toes forward as far as you can, then bring your toes back towards you. Work your way up to 30 repetitions. With this dynamic stretching routine, you are stretching the front and back of your calf musculature. Once you are done with the left side, perform the same thing on the right.

8

Applying These Principles Away From the Desk

I've provided ways to attain the correct postures, but I want to make sure that you realize you should always try to maintain these postures when you're away from your desk, regardless of what you are doing. I want to discuss a few instances when you may be stuck in a seated position for a long period of time and how you can try to minimize the pain associated with them. Some common instances when you might be in a prolonged sitting position outside of the office may be waiting rooms, airplanes, and car rides.

First off, let's begin with waiting rooms. I bring up waiting rooms because, in my experience, the time we spend waiting in these settings can vary. It is important that, if you're waiting for a long period of time, you try to stand up and walk around just like I suggested earlier. The furniture in waiting areas can vary, so I cannot say with certainty that they will be an ideal size for you. Stand up, walk around, just try to not sit dormant for a long period of time because your posture will break eventually.

During a car ride, you should adjust your seat as best you can to fit with the instructions I outlined earlier. While in the car, try to maintain your optimal upper and lower body positioning. I really like the idea of stopping every hour or so (I know that you may not want to stop every 50 minutes). If you cannot do this, then try to stop as much as you are allowed to. Most people like to fall asleep when they're passengers during a car ride, so I suggest using pillows and things to help keep you upright in the correct posture. Play around with placement to fit it correctly for you. While riding in the car, you can perform some of the exercises I have outlined earlier. I would suggest performing the neck stretches and chin tucks whenever you start to feel discomfort. The scapular squeezes will also help you get out of the rounded shoulder posture. If you are the driver during this long trip, try to do some repetitions during red lights or while sitting completely still in traffic. Doing exercises while moving is UNSAFE, and I advise against it.

During a trip on an airplane, you have more options than in a car. First off, you can usually walk around and stand up when the captain and crew clear you to. This is important, especially on very long flights, because postures tend to get very bad on long flights. You've probably seen people hunched over the tray while sleeping or using their portable devices in extremely slouched postures. This is primarily due to the tray being so low. Unfortunately, it cannot be adjusted, so if you want to use your mobile device, try to place something underneath to bring it upwards. I've seen some pretty impressive devices that allow you to mount your tablet and/or phone to eye level, which could be a viable option. I would also suggest trying to perform the scapular squeezes, chin tucks, and neck stretches when necessary. If you find room, try to perform some of the lower body stretching outlined before.

In the classroom, posture can also take a toll because we are sitting for long lectures, taking tests, and are sometimes bored out of our minds. Do not let your posture suffer because of this environment! In the classroom, some bad postures I have seen include the laptop position I talked about earlier, head resting on hands, and just overall slouching forward. Remember to try to implement the methods I discussed earlier. If you happen to get distracted, try to correct your posture as much as possible.

9

Epilogue

I've given you some key strategies to stay pain-free at your desk and I've provided you with other real-life examples of when they can be applied. It is important to try and implement these as soon as possible because you don't want to maintain bad habits when it comes to your posture. Take it from me, I have treated a lot of people so far in my career and a good number of them have had very poor posture. Sure, accidents happen and injuries occur, but implementing optimal posture strategies will decrease your chances of becoming injured and experiencing pain. Maintain that proper foundation to your house and you should be able to keep it very stable.

After you begin to implement these optimal posture strategies, you will begin to notice people throughout the course of your day doing the wrong thing. With the examples I have given, you will also be able to discover ways to help maintain a good posture in nearly every situation. Following this guideline in everything you do should help decrease the amount of time you experience discomfort and allow you to enjoy a pain-free life. I want to thank you for your time, and I wish you the best of luck in maintaining optimal posture!

References

Houglum, P. Therapeutic Exercises for Musculoskeletal Injuries.

Nejati P., Lotfian S., Moezy A., Nejati M. The Study of Correlation Between Forward Head Posture and Neck Pain in Iranian Office Workers. *International Journal of Occupational Medicine and Environmental Health*. 2015; 28(2): 295-303. doi:10.13075/ijomeh.1896.00352

Jung S.I., Lee N.K., Kang K.W., Kim K., Lee D.Y. The Effect of Smartphone Usage Time on Posture and Respiratory Function. *Journal of Physical Therapy Science*. 2016; 28(1): 186-189. doi:10.1589/jpts.28.186.

Kim D., Cho M., Park Y., Yang Y. Effect of an Exercise Program for Posture Correction on Musculoskeletal Pain. *Journal of Physical Therapy Science*. 2015; 27(6): 1791-1794. doi:10.1589/jpts.27.1791.

About the Author

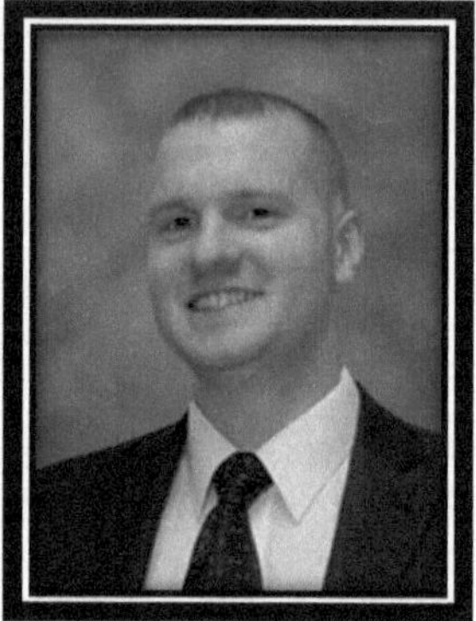

Nicholas Gallo is a board certified Doctor of Physical Therapy. He has helped countless patients in his career and continues to practice Physical Therapy on a full time basis. He is also a cofounder of Physical Therapy 101.

Additional Resources

For more information, visit my website at www.physicaltherapy101.net. Here we have resources on various pathologies. This website is continuously updated to provide up to date treatment.

Subscribe to my YouTube channel https://www.youtube.com/c/PhysicalTherapy101. Here we produce free treatment videos for patients and healthcare providers. This is also a great visual aid for treatments described above.

P.S. If you have enjoyed this book and found it resourceful, please leave a helpful review on Amazon.